Medication Technician Study Guide

Medication Aide Training Manual

Jane John-Nwankwo   RN, MSN

MEDICATION TECHNICIAN STUDY GUIDE:
Medication Aide Training Manual

ISBN-13: 978-1533497062

ISBN-10: 1533497060

Printed in the United States of America.

Have you bought these books?

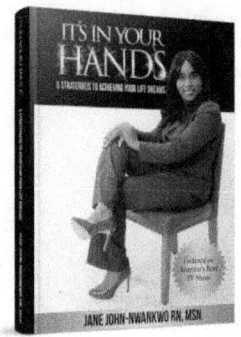

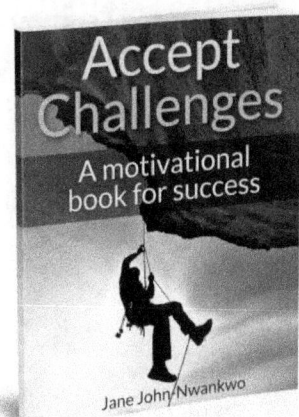

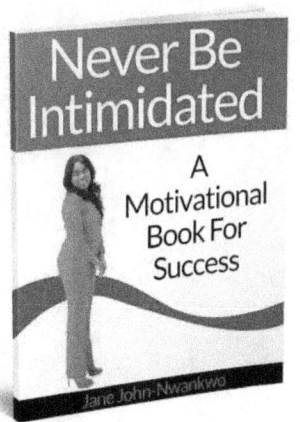

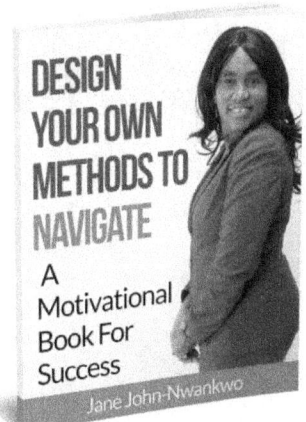

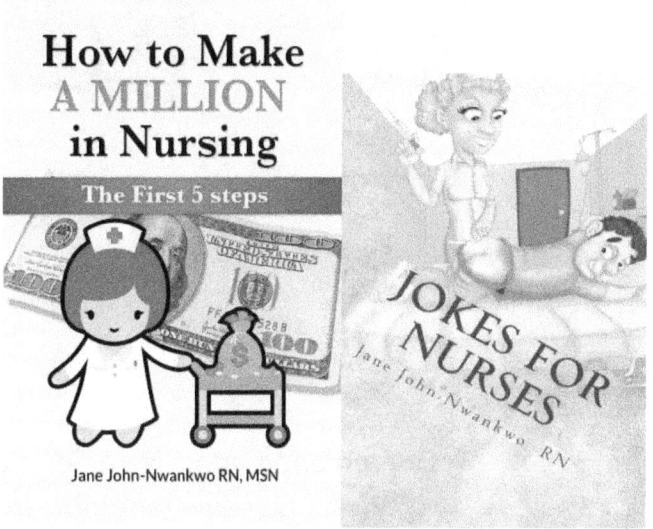

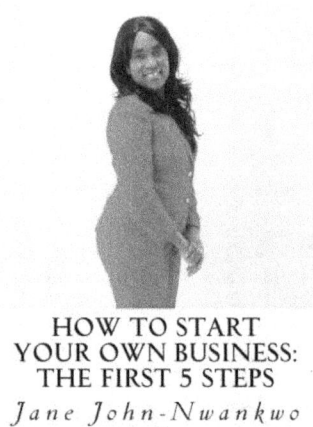

HOW TO START
YOUR OWN BUSINESS:
THE FIRST 5 STEPS
Jane John-Nwankwo

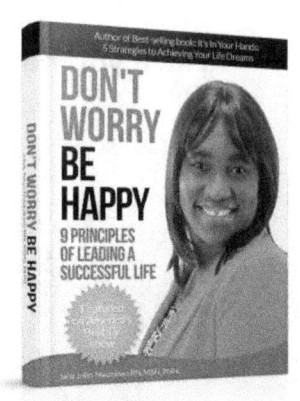

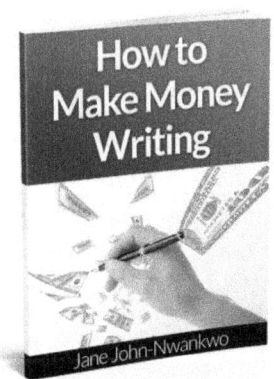

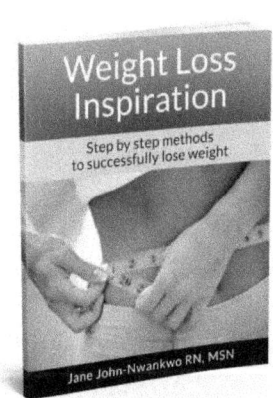

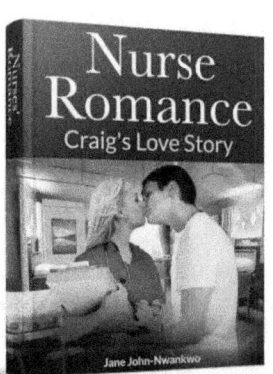

Search Jane John-Nwankwo on Amazon.com
Website: www.janejohn-nwankwo.com

Dedication

To my loving daughter, Jessica.

THINGS YOU WILL LEARN FROM THIS BOOK

Who is a medication technician or medication aide.

Responsibilities of a medication aide.

Vital Signs.

History of medications and medication administration.

Principles of Medication Administration.

Different Routes of medication administrations.

Drugs affecting the cardiovascular system.

Drugs affecting the urinary system.

Drugs affecting the respiratory system.

Drugs affecting the digestive system, vitamins, and minerals.

Drugs affecting the central nervous system.

Affecting the musculoskeletal system.

Drugs affecting the endocrine system.

Antibiotics and other anti-infective agents .

Drugs affecting the eye.

Drugs affecting the ear.

The Medication Technician

Introduction

In hospitals and healthcare settings, there is a high requirement for capable personnel who can distribute and administer medications to patients. Such personnel are required in hospitals, nursing facilities, correctional institutions, assisted living homes, clinics and other similar healthcare institutions. In order to meet this demand, a whole new job role has emerged – that of a medication technician or medication aide. In order to become a medication technician, a short training course along with a test certification is mandatory according to state laws (French and Fordney, 2012). Medication technicians are also referred to as medication aides, medication assistants, certified residential care medication aide, medication assistive person, registered medication aide, medication aide credentialed, qualified medication aide, etc. The duties of medication aides are determined according to the medical practice act of every state. It is not required for medical assistants working under the direct supervision of a physician to become a medication technician in order to be able to administer medication.

Functions of a Medication Technician

A medication technician is involved in distributing and administering medications to patients. They usually work under doctoral or nursing supervision. They assist patients in consuming medications topically or orally. They are required to follow strict medical protocol and administer correct dosages in the right manner. They are also required to monitor patients to make sure that no adverse reactions are occurring unnoticed. The complete medication history and medication records of patients have to be maintained by medication technicians for each medication that has been administered (Durgin and Hanan, 2004).

A medication technician is required to know the proper methodology of administering different kinds of medications, whether they are administered topically, orally, vaginally, rectally or transdermally. They should also possess knowledge on medication administration through nebulizers, inhalers and tubes. They are however restricted from administering injections, whether intravenously, intradermally or intramuscularly.

Basic Requirements

Medication technicians administering medications to patients should be free of communicable infections such as sore throat, cold or open lesions (Durgin and Hanan, 2004). This requirement is of importance, both for the drug administrator and the patient. Patients are often susceptible to acquiring nosocomial infections as they are weak and because their immune system could be compromised because of radiation therapy, surgery and other such procedures or other reasons such as diseases, malnutrition or ageing.

Drug administrators who are in poor health or are exhausted are more likely to commit errors in medication administration, unlike those who are alert, attentive and in good health. Healthcare professionals are more susceptible to acquiring infections from patients if they are in poor health. As medication technicians are involved in direct care of patients and drug administration, they are required to maintain their health through healthy living habits, diet and exercise. If afflicted with an upper respiratory infection or other communicable diseases, medication technicians should inform their supervisors so arrangements can be made to avoid tasks that involve direct patient care until they are back in good health. Medication technicians should also possess knowledge in using appropriate protective devices during medication administration to avoid disease transmission, especially blood borne. In case of isolated patients with infectious diseases, hospital policies on protection need to be followed. They are also required to be aware of basic safety protocols, aseptic techniques and hospital protocols concerning safety measures, for both healthcare personnel and patients.

Difference between Medication Aide and Medication Technician – Historical Development

The terms 'medication technician' and 'medication aide' are often used interchangeably. However, there are some basic differences between the two. The role of a 'medication assistant' was created when the Health Occupations Article Title 8-6A-01 et. seq. law was passed in 1998 that required the certification of nursing assistants (Maryland Board of Nursing, 2008). The definition of a medication assistant was given as "an individual who completes a Board approved 16 hour Medication Administration Training Program" (Maryland Board of Nursing, 2008). Medication assistants were required by law to be registered with the Board of Nursing. Upon registration, they could administer certain medications to patients in selected community settings under two circumstances – when delegated to do so by a registered nurse, and when the administration was done under the direct supervision, instruction and evaluation of a registered nurse. Medication assistants could function in certain settings such as a Developmental Disabilities alternative living unit, assisted living institution, schools, and residential placement programs of the Department of Juvenile Service.

To be eligible for the Medication Assistant Training Program approved by the board, an individual was required to be employed in a healthcare setting and a recommendation from his/her employer was required. Nursing Assistant Certification was not mandatory for becoming a medication assistant. After the passing of a new legislation SB405 in 2004, medication assistants were certified under a new title of the 'Medication Technician'. This legislation also laid down the minimum age limit for working as a medication technician and the hours of training were increased to 20 hours from the previous 16 hours. Disciplinary action to be taken against medication technicians in case of faults was also defined by this legislation.

Certified medication technicians are different from certified medication aides. The Certified Medicine Aide (CMA) job role has existed since 1970s and is regulated under the COMAR (Code of Maryland Regulation) 10.07.02. To be able to work as a medication aide, the individual should hold an active CNA (Certified Nursing Assistant) certification. Medication aides carry out medication administration and nursing functions under the supervision of a licensed nurse. The functions, responsibilities and requirements are different for both medication aides and medication technicians. Therefore, these are two separate professional entities. However, in most states, Medication Technicians and Medication aides are brought under a single role.

Responsibilities of a Medication Technician

The role of a medication technician (MT) is that of extremely high responsibility. A medication technician should be able to appreciate the inherent responsibility of his role in a healthcare setting. In addition, an MT should also be knowledgeable about the roles and responsibilities of the other members of his health team, especially in relation to the communication involved with drug administration.

He should give high priority to care of patients and should treat each one of them with professional concern and dignity (Durgin and Hanan, 2004). He should treat patients well regardless of their mental or physical impairment, cultural background, race, lifestyle orientation or religious beliefs.

He should be thorough in procedures and policies that dictate medical protocol in hospitals. He should also know the pharmacist, physician and nurse to whom he reports directly. He is also required to report any unusual changes, be they emotional or physical, noted at the time of medication rounds to the nurse in charge. He is also required to maintain professional confidentiality about the patients in his care. MTs need to report to work in professional attire with their identification badge held in place.

The prime responsibility of an MT is to administer daily medications to patients. They are also required to observe patients closely to report any adverse drug effects. They monitor the vital signs of patients, calculate the medication dosages and record the medication history and progress of patients. Before administering drugs to patients, medication technicians should be aware of the general uses and indications of the drug, the dosage range and usual dose of the drug, special precautions to be taken for each drug, side effects that may occur upon drug administration, foods or drugs that cannot be given along with a specific drug and the time when onset of drug action is expected (Durgin and Hanan, 2004).

The roles and responsibilities of MTs have been explicitly stated out according to state laws. The responsibility of an MT is to assist a licensed nurse in providing ethical and safe care to patients (by administering prescribed medications and completing other nursing tasks that are allowed by state law. Some of the main responsibilities of an MT according to Whitenton and Walker, 2013, are:

-functions as a member of a healthcare team

-carries out tasks associated with nursing assistance

- assists nurses in providing care to patients that also includes observing and reporting the needs of the patient.

- recognizes and performs tasks as per his level of training and education.

- accepts accountability and responsibility of his own performance as per the regulations and state laws governing his role.

- carries out his tasks in a caring, ethical and legal manner; informs supervisors about changes in the status of a patient; creates documents as per the standard policies

-carries out his tasks safely to ensure comfort and welfare of patients

- respects the rights of patients; protects the confidential information of his patients unless otherwise required for the welfare and safety of the patient

- follows all the state and federal regulations for the protection of his own and others' health; and takes guidance from nurse as and when needed in order to carry out his tasks efficiently and safely.

The job duties and responsibilities of an MT include the administration of scheduled drugs under the direct supervision of a licensed nurse or without the supervision if allowed under a state law; giving the PRN medications as needed; carrying out tasks that are associated with administration of medication, such as checking vital signs, monitoring glucose, measuring weight and height, and observing patients; recording the administration of medication as per the procedure of the agency; reporting patient status changes in response to drug therapy; reporting any events that may be life-threatening to ensure the safety of himself, the patient and others; and reporting errors in medication administration and drugs and filling out the appropriate forms (Whitenton and Walker, 2013).

MTs do have some role limitations that are legally binding. For instance, they cannot give the first dose of a medication that is newly ordered, they are not given medications that require conversion of dosage from one measurement method to another, they are not required to give medications in case of nurse unavailability for monitoring the effects of the medications on patients, they are not given the liberty to take their own decisions that may include the withholding of a medication, they cannot be delegated with functions that involve the regulation of IV fluids, programming of insulin or IV pumps and the administration of drugs to unstable patients, and they are also not required to administer medications nasogastrically, parenterally, through jejunostomy or through gastrostomy (Whitenton and Walker, 2013). The limitations however vary regionally and as per state laws applicable.

MTs need to be knowledgeable about basic pharmacology and the principles of medication administration. Their clinical competencies include – knowing the rights of medication administration, understanding when to accept a delegation for administration of a medication and when to decline it, documenting the administration of a medication accurately, and notifying the nurse in charge about the patient's condition (Cima, 2011).

Vital Signs

Reflect the functions of three body processes necessary for life:

Body temperature

Respiration

Heart function

The four vital signs of body function are:

Temperature

Pulse

Respiration

Blood pressure

Temperature

Body temperature is a balance between heat production and heat loss in conjunction with each other, maintained and regulated by the hypothalamus.

Thermometers are used to measure temperature using the Fahrenheit and Centigrade or Celsius scale. Temperature sites are the following: mouth, rectum, ear (tympanic membrane), and the axilla (underarm). The normal ranges for each site are:

Site	Normal Range
Rectal	98.6Fto 100.6F (37.0C to 38.1C)

Oral	97.6F to 99.6F (36.5C to 37.5C)
Axillary	96.6F to 98.6F (35.9C to 37.0C)
Tympanic Membrane	98.6F (37C)

Some terms used to describe body temperature are:

Febrile – presence of fever

Afebrile – absence of fever

Fever – elevated body temperature beyond normal range. Types of fever are:

Intermittent: fluctuating fever that returns to or below baseline then rises again.

Remittent: fluctuating fever that remains elevated; it does not return to baseline temperature.

Continuous: a fever that remains constant above the baseline; it does not fluctuate.

Oral temperature is the most common method of measurement; however, it is not taken from the following patients:

- infants and children less than six years old

- patients who has had surgery or facial, neck, nose, or mouth injury

- those receiving oxygen

- those with nasogastric tubes

- patients with convulsive seizure

- hemiplegic patients

- patients with altered mental status

Wait for 30 minutes to take the oral temperature in patients who have just finished eating, drinking, or smoking. When taking the temperature, leave the thermometer in the patient's mouth for 3-5 minutes or as required by agency policy.

Rectal temperature is taken when oral temperature is not feasible. However, it is not taken from the following patients:

- patients with heart disease

- patients with rectal disease or disorder or has had rectal surgery

- patients with diarrhea

It is taken with the patient in a side-lying position and the thermometer and the patient's hip is held throughout the procedure so the thermometer is not lost in the rectum or broken.

Axillary temperature is the least accurate and is taken only when no other temperature site can be used. The axilla, (the underarm) should be clean and dry and the thermometer should be held in place for 5-10 minutes or as required by the facility policy.

Tympanic temperature is useful for children and confused patients because of the speed of operation of the tympanic thermometer. A covered probe is gently inserted into the ear canal and temperature is measured within seconds (1–3 seconds). It is not used if the patient has an ear disorder or ear drainage.

Pulse

The normal adult pulse rate ranges between 60 and 100 beats per minute. The site most commonly used for taking pulse is the radial artery found in the wrist on the same side as the thumb. It is felt with the first two or three fingers (never with the thumb) and usually taken for 30 seconds multiplied by two to get the rate per minute. If the rate is unusually fast or slow, however, count it for 60 seconds.

The apical pulse is a more accurate measurement of the heart rate and it is taken over the apex of the heart by auscultation using the stethoscope. It is used for patients with irregular heart rate and for infants and small children.

Respiration

When measuring respiration, respiratory characteristics such as rate, rhythm, and depth are taken into account. Rate is the number of respirations per minute. The normal range for adults is 12 to 20 per minute. One inspiration (inhalation) and one expiration (exhalation) counts as one respiration. It is counted for 30 seconds multiplied by two or for a full minute.

Some rate abnormalities are the following:

Apnea – this is a temporary complete absence of breathing which may be a result of a

reduction in the stimuli to the respiratory centers of the brain.

Tachypnea – this is a respiration rate of greater than 40/min. It is transient in the newborn and maybe caused by the hysteria in the adult.

Bradypnea – decrease in numbers of respirations. This occurs during sleep. It may also

be due to certain diseases.

Respiratory rhythm refers to the pattern of breathing. It can vary with age: infants have an irregular rhythm while adults have regular.

Some abnormalities in the rhythm are the following:

Cheyne-Stokes – this is a regular pattern of irregular breathing rate.

Orthopnea – this is difficulty or inability to breath unless in an upright position.

Depth of respiration refers to the amount of air that is inspired and expired during each

respiration. Some abnormalities in the depth of respirations are the following:

Hypoventilation: state in which reduced amount of air enters the lungs resulting in decreased oxygen level and increased carbon dioxide level in blood. It can be due to breathing that is too shallow, or too slow, or to diminished lung function.

Hyperpnea: abnormal increase in the depth and rate of breathing.

Hyperventilation: state in which there is an increased amount of air entering the lungs.

Blood Pressure

This is the measurement of the amount of force exerted by the blood on the peripheral arterial walls and is expressed in millimeters (mm) of mercury (Hg).The measurement consist of two components: the highest (systole) and lowest (diastole) amount of pressure exerted during the cardiac cycle.

A stethoscope and sphygmomanometer of either aneroid or mercury type are used. The size of the cuff of the sphygmomanometer will depend on the circumference of the limb and not the age of the patient. The width of the inflatable bag within the cuff should be about 40% of this circumference – 12 cm to 14 cm in an average adult. The length of the bag should be about 80% of this circumference – almost long enough to encircle the arm. Cuffs that are too short or narrow may give falsely high readings, e.g. a regular cuff on an obese arm may lead to a false diagnosis of hypertension.

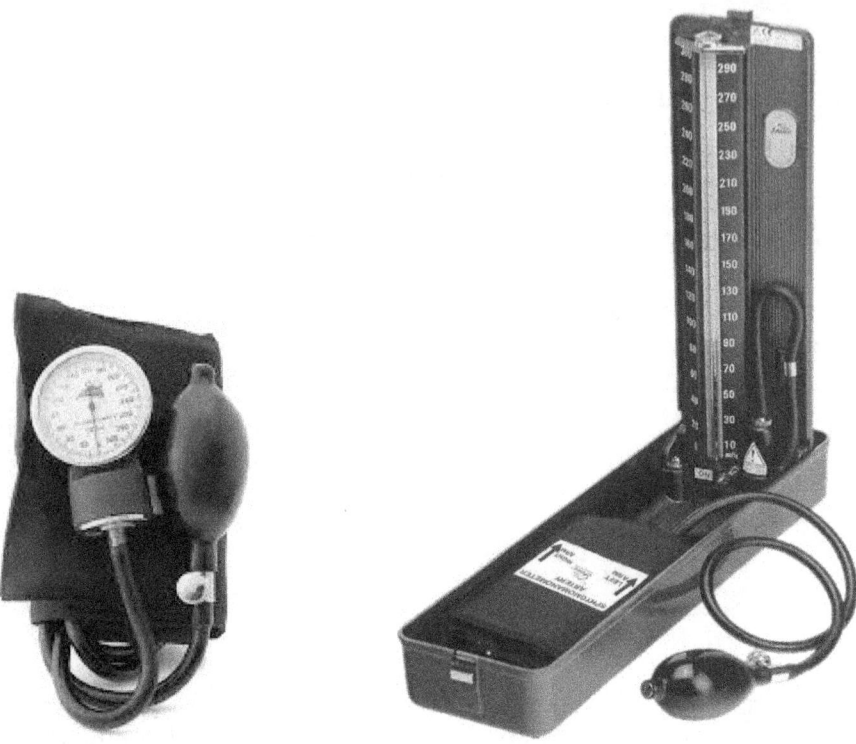

The inflatable bag is centered over the brachial artery with the lower border about 2.5cm above the antecubital crease. The cuff is positioned at heart level. If the brachial artery is far below the heart level the blood pressure will appear falsely high. If the brachial artery is far above heart level, blood pressure will appear falsely low.

Blood pressure is taken by determining first the palpatory systolic pressure over the brachial artery. Then with the bell of the stethoscope over the brachial artery, the cuff is inflated again to about 30 mm Hg above the palpatory systolic pressure and deflated slowly, allowing the pressure to drop at a rate of about 2 to 3 mmHg per second. Note the level at which you hear the sounds of at least two consecutive beats. This is the systolic pressure. Continue to lower the pressure slowly until the sounds become muffled and then disappear. Then deflate the cuff rapidly to zero. The disappearance point, which is usually only a few mmHg below the muffling point, marks the generally accepted diastolic pressure. Both the systolic and diastolic pressure levels are read the nearest 2 mmHg.

Common errors in blood pressure measurements:

Improper cuff size. Cuffs that are too short or narrow may give falsely high readings. Using a regular cuff on an obese arm may lead to a false diagnosis of hypertension. For an obese arm, select a cuff with a larger than standard bag.

The arm is not at heart level. If the brachial artery is much below the heart level, the blood pressure will appear falsely high. Conversely, if the artery is much above heart level, blood pressure will appear falsely low. A 13.6 cm difference between arterial and cardiac levels produces a blood pressure error of 10mmHg.

Cuff is not completely deflated before use. Deflation of the cuff is faster than 2-3 mmHg per second. Rapid deflation will lead to underestimation of the systolic and overestimation of the diastolic pressure.

The cuff is re-inflated during the procedure without allowing the arm to rest for 1-2 minute between readings. Repetitive inflation of the cuff can result in venous congestion, which could make the sound less audible producing artificially low systolic and high diastolic pressure.

Improper cuff placement.

Defective equipment. A bag that balloons outside the cuff leads to falsely high readings.

Anthropometric Measurements

The term anthropometric refers to comparative measurements of the body. They are used as indicators of the state of health and well-being of the patient and are often included in the initial measurement of vital signs. Anthropometric measurements require precise measuring techniques to be valid.

Length, height, weight, weight-for-length, and head circumference (length is used in infants and toddlers, rather than height, because they are unable to stand) are used to assess growth and development in infants, children and adolescents. Individual measurements are usually compared to reference standards on a growth chart.

Height, weight, body mass index (BMI), waist-to-hip ratio, and percentage of body fat are the measurements used for adults. These measures are then compared to reference standards to assess weight status and the risk for various diseases.

History of Medications and Medication Administration

In a healthcare setting, documenting medication histories is extremely crucial in order to avoid prescription errors and risks to patients. Apart from the prevention of prescription errors, taking down medication histories accurately is helpful in detecting any changes in clinical signs or drug-related pathology (FitzGerald, 2009). A well-documented medication history includes all the prescribed drugs, all earlier adverse drug reactions and herbal/alternative medicines in addition to any over-the-counter medications taken by the patient. It also reports the patient's adherence to therapy.

Importance of Medication History

MTs are required to take down accurate medication history. This is because knowing what drugs a patient has taken in the past and the present, and his/her responses to these drugs enables a better planning of future treatment (FitzGerald, 2009). Drugs can also result in diseases and illnesses thus, the effects of drugs should always be included in differential diagnoses reports. Another reason for taking down medication history is that drugs cannot only mask clinical signs but also alter the results of investigations. Therefore, any subsequent results of drug administration can be acted upon by knowing which drugs have been used. The medication history can also be used to inform the patients about their prescriptions and to help in the avoidance of preventable errors that may occur during prescription.

The medication history of a patient must not simply be a list of the drugs and dosage administered to a patient but should include information such as previous and current hypersensitivity reactions if any, adherence to therapy, and adverse effects. This data needs to be reported and compared with general medical records of the patient or the previous history of prescriptions given to the patient. It is often seen that adverse drug reactions are not recorded properly (FitzGerald, 2009). Moreover, herbal remedies taken by patients are also not recorded most times. These could be crucial causes of morbidity and cannot be ignored.

For instance, as described by Constable et al. (cited in FitzGerald, 2009), a 77-year old female patient on a lansoprazole prescription suffered from upper gastrointestinal haemorrhage after the induction of CYP2C19 through the use of St John's wort in addition to platelet aggregation inhibition because of the use of ginseng. None of these herbal medications were reported in the admission drug history of the patient, although these were extremely involved in the presentation and could influence further episodes of the condition. In addition to herbal medications, many types of complementary and alternative medicine (CAM) are either not recorded or are recorded improperly.

Reporting of a Good Medication History

According to FitzGerald (2009), a good medication history should elicit all information associated with any kind of drug or therapy use. A medication history should use the word medication or medicines instead of 'drugs' as the use of the word drug may be misconstrued as drugs of abuse. A good patient history of medication administration should describe and report the current prescribed formulations, drugs, routes of administration, dosage, duration of treatment and frequency. Other medications such as herbal, natural or over-the-counter medicines should be aptly recorded. Any drugs that have been administered in the recent past, previous hypersensitivity reactions to drugs, their time course and nature, previous adverse drug reactions, their time course and nature and the patient's adherence to therapy also need to be recorded.

History from a community pharmacist or a general practitioner needs to have an updated list of medications, dates when medications were last ordered and the previous adverse reactions to drugs. History derived from case notes needs to have details concerning previous prescriptions and the previous adverse reactions to drugs. The containers of medications and the medications themselves need to be examined for dosage, name and the amount of dosage forms taken since the dispensing of the drug. Merely by inspecting the formulation, it is possible to identify a medication (FitzGerald, 2009).

Safety

Safety hazards abound in the healthcare setting, many of which can cause serious injury or disease. The Occupational Safety and Health Administration (OSHA) is responsible for the identification of the various hazards present in the workplace and for the creation of rules and regulations to minimize exposure to such hazards. Employers are mandated to institute measures that will assure safe working conditions and health workers have the obligation to know and follow those measures.

Safety rules are usually based on common sense. Most accidents occur when these rules are neglected, overlooked or ignored. Accidents generally occur when safety is compromised because of haste and secondary shortcuts. These shortcuts can lead to personal injury and equipment damage. When an accident occurs, it must be reported to your supervisor immediately. Trying to cover up the incident can lead to serious, even disastrous results.

Hazards

A. Physical Hazards

Electrical Safety Regulations

Use only ground plugs that have been approved by Underwriters' Laboratory (UL).

Never use extension cords.

Avoid electrical circuit overloading.

Inspect all cords and plugs periodically for damage.

Use a surge protector on all sensitive electronic devices.

Before servicing, UNPLUG the device from the electrical outlet.

Use signs and/or labels to indicate high voltage or electrical hazards.

B. Chemical Hazards

Chemical Safety Regulations

If the skin or eyes come in contact with any chemicals, immediately wash the area with water for at least 5 minutes.

Store flammable or volatile chemicals in a well-ventilated area.

After use, immediately recap all bottles containing toxic substances.

Label all chemicals with the required Material Safety Data Sheet (MDSD) information.

C. Biological Hazards

Biological Safety Regulations

1. Disinfect the laboratory work area before and after each use when dealing with biologicals.

2. Never draw a specimen through a pipette by mouth. This technique is not permitted in the laboratory.

3. Always wear gloves.

4. Sterilize specimens and any other contaminated materials and/or dispose of them through incineration.

5. Wash hands thoroughly before and after every procedure.

Emergency First Aid

The ability to recognize and react quickly to an emergency may be the difference of life or death for the patient. As patients react differently to various situations, it is important for all healthcare professionals to be prepared in an emergency.

External Hemorrhage: controlling the bleeding is most effectively accomplished by elevating the affected part above heart level and applying direct pressure to the wound. Do not attempt to elevate a broken extremity as this could cause further damage.

Shock occurs when there is _insufficient return of blood flow to the heart, resulting in inadequate supply of oxygen to all organs and tissues of the body.' Patients experiencing trauma may go into shock and for some patients, seeing their own blood may induce shock.

Common symptoms:

-Pale, cold, clammy skin

-Rapid, weak pulse

- Increased, shallow breathing rate

- Expressionless face/staring eyes.

First Aid for Shock:

-Maintain an open airway for the victim

-Call for assistance

-Keep the victim lying down with the head lower than the rest of the body

-Attempt to control bleeding or cause of shock (if known)

-Keep the victim warm until help arrives

Cardiopulmonary Resuscitation. Most healthcare institutions require their professionals to be certified in CPR. It is important for all professionals to maintain all certifications acquired.

Infection Control/Chain of Infection

This consists of links, each of which is necessary for the infectious disease to spread. Infection control is based on the fact that the transmission of infectious diseases will be prevented or stopped when any level in the chain is broken or interrupted.

Agent -------------- Mode of transmission ------------ Susceptible host

: :

: :

portal of exit portal of entry

Agents– are infectious microorganisms that can be classified into groups namely: viruses, bacteria, fungi, and parasites. When infectious diseases are identified according to the specific disease-causing microorganism, the disease may be prevented with the use of anti-infective drugs or infection control practices.

Portal of exit –the method by which an infectious agent leaves its reservoir. Standard

Precautions and Transmission-Based Precautions are control measures aimed at

preventing the spread of the disease as infectious agents exit the reservoir.

Mode of transmission –specific ways in which microorganisms travel from the reservoir

to the susceptible host. There are five main types of mode of transmission:

- Contact : direct and indirect

- Droplet

- Airborne

- Common vehicle

- Vectorborne

Portal of entry – allows the infectious agent access to the susceptible host. Common

entry sites are broken skin, mucous membranes, and body systems exposed to the

external environment such as the respiratory, gastrointestinal, and reproductive. Methods such as sterile

wound care, transmission-based precautions, and aseptic technique limit the transmission of the

infectious agents.

Susceptible host – The infectious agent enters a person who is not resistant or immune.

Control at this level is directed towards the identification of the patients at risk, treat their underlying

condition for susceptibility, or isolate them from the reservoir.

Medical Asepsis

Best defined as —the destruction of pathogenic microorganisms after they leave the body.‖ It also

involves environmental hygiene measures such as equipment cleaning and disinfection procedures.

Methods of medical asepsis are Standard Precautions and Transmission-Based Precautions

Disinfection. This procedure used in medical asepsis using various chemicals that can be used to destroy

many pathogenic microorganisms. Since chemicals can irritate skin and mucous membranes, they are

used only on inanimate objects.

The least expensive and most readily available disinfectant for surfaces such as

countertops is a 1:10 solution of household bleach. Boiling water (temperature of 212 F)

is considered a form of disinfection, but use of it in today's medical setting is limited to

items that:

1. will not be used in invasive procedures;

2. will not be inserted into body orifices nor be used in a sterile procedure

Surgical Asepsis

All microbial life, pathogens and nonpathogens, are destroyed before an invasive procedure is performed. Surgical asepsis and sterile technique are often used interchangeably.

Four methods of sterilization

1. Gas sterilization: often used for wheelchairs and hospital beds. Useful in hospitals, but costly for the office.

2. Dry heat sterilization: requires higher temperature that steam sterilization but longer exposure times. Used for instruments that easily corrodes.

3. Chemical sterilization - uses the same chemical used for chemical disinfection, but the exposure time is longer.

4. Steam sterilization (autoclave) - uses steam under pressure to obtain high temperature of 250-254F with exposure times of 20-40 minutes depending on the item being sterilized.

Handwashing

Hand washing is the most important means of preventing the spread of infection. A routine hand wash procedure uses plain soap to remove soil and transient bacteria. Hand antisepsis requires the use of antimicrobial soap to remove, kill or inhibit transient microorganisms. It is important that all healthcare personnel learn proper hand washing procedures.

Barrier Protection

Protective clothing provides a barrier against infection. Used properly, it will provide protection to the person wearing it; disposed of properly it will assist in the spread of infection. Learning how to put on and remove protective clothing is vital to insure the health and wellness of the person wearing the PPE. PPE's or personal protective equipment includes:

Masks

Goggles

Face Shields

Respirator

Isolation Precautions

For many years, the CDC recommended universal precautions, which is a method of infection control that assumed that all human blood and body fluids were potentially infectious. The CDC issued a revised guidelines consisting of two tiers or levels of precautions: Standard Precautions and Transmission-Based Precautions.

Standard Precautions

This is an infection control method designed to prevent direct contact with blood and

other body fluids and tissues by using barrier protection and work control practices.

Under the standard precautions, all patients are presumed to be infective for blood-borne pathogens. Infection control practices to be used with all patients. These replace universal precautions and body substance isolation. They are used when there is a possibility of contact with any of the following:

- Blood

- All body fluids, secretions, and excretions (except sweat), regardless of whether or not they contain visible blood

- Nonintact skin

- Mucous membranes designed to reduce the risk of transmission of microorganisms from both

- Recognized and unrecognized sources of infections.

The standard precautions are:

Wear gloves when collecting and handling blood, body fluids, or tissue specimen. Wear face shields when there is a danger for splashing on mucous membranes. Dispose of all needles and sharp objects in puncture-proof containers without recapping.

Transmission- Based Precautions the second tier of precautions and are to be used when the patient is known or suspected of being infected with contagious disease. They are to be used in addition to standard precautions. All types of isolation are condensed into three categories:

Contact precautions: are designed to reduce the risk of transmission of microorganisms by direct or indirect contact. Direct-contact transmission involves skin-to-skin contact and physical transfer of microorganisms to a susceptible host from an infected or colonized person. Indirect-contact

transmission involves contact with a contaminated intermediate object in the patient's environment

Airborne precautions: are designed to reduce the risk of airborne transmission of infectious agents. Microorganisms carried in this manner can be dispersed widely by air currents and may become inhaled by or deposited on a susceptible host within the same room or over a longer distance from the source patient. Special air handling and ventilation are required to prevent airborne transmission.

Contact precautions: are designed to reduce the risk of transmission of microorganisms by direct or indirect contact. Direct-contact transmission involves skin-to-skin contact and physical transfer of microorganisms to a susceptible host from an infected or colonized person. Indirect-contact

transmission involves contact with a contaminated intermediate object in the patient's environment

Airborne precautions: are designed to reduce the risk of airborne transmission of infectious agents. Microorganisms carried in this manner can be dispersed widely by air currents and may become inhaled by or deposited on a susceptible host within the same room or over a longer distance from the source patient. Special air handling and ventilation are required to prevent airborne transmission.

Errors in Medication History

There has been a tremendous amount of research on medication errors, beginning with a study that established the fact that medication errors are a much bigger problem than was actually realized (Flynn, n.d.). Errors in medication administration were employed by researchers to study the output quality of drug distribution systems in the 1960s at the time of development of the unit dose drug distribution system. These errors were considered an important indicator of drug therapy quality for the patient. Research on devices that perform automatic drug dispensing has shown that errors are still a common occurrence (Flynn, n.d.). Errors of medication history, such as the omission of drugs, are common. These errors can bring harm to the patient. Moreover, hypersensitivity reactions are not explored in detail or are improperly documented, which may help in a drug being avoided unnecessarily. In addition, clinical specialty, specific drugs and polypharmacy can influence the risks of errors in medication history. Some of the reasons for the common occurrence of medication errors upon admission to hospitals include the inability of patients to accurately report their drug history. They also do not bring their previous medications or a list of those medications along with them (FitzGerald, 2009).

Principles of Medication Administration

Regardless of the type of medication, certain basic principles dictate the process of medication administration. As part of these principles, MTs are required to talk to their patients and communicate what will be done before the medication is administered. Any question that the patient may have should be clearly addressed by the professional or directed to the licensed nurse overshadowing them. They need to help the patients in getting involved in the process of medication administration. They also need to provide privacy to the patients. The process of medication administration should be given complete and undivided attention and should be carried out in an area that is free from distraction. MTs need to maintain cleanliness and hygiene, and should wash their hands prior to and after the administration of medication. Clayton (2012) elaborated the principles of medication administration and safety as follows:

Standards of Care, Basic Requirements and Patient Charts

The standards of care are developed by state as well as federal law in addition to the Joint Commission and professional organizations involved in patient care and treatment. MTs are required to be familiar with the contents of the nurse practice act and any legislation that dictates their profession. The law of each state has certain limitations regarding the administration of medication. Separate policies are also provided by the healthcare institutions. Knowing and following these are the duties of MTs and all other professionals.

While administering a medication, an MT should have the certification and permission to practice, and a policy statement authorizing the act. He should understand the patient's symptoms and diagnosis that correlate with the rationale of the administration of the medication. He should know why the particular drug administration has been ordered, its expected outcome, dilution, dosing, rate of administration, route of administration, expected adverse effects and contraindications.

He should also be able to calculate, prepare and administer the drug accurately, apart from assessing the patient to detect any therapeutic or adverse effect the medication may have induced. The professional administering the medication should actively participate in educating the family of the patient and the patient himself regarding the treatment and discharge of the patient. In many states, this is the duty of the registered or Licensed Vocational Nurse.

Patient charts are records that provide information to all the healthcare team members about the status of the patient, his progress and care. These are legal documents that not only describe his health but also list all the therapeutic and diagnostic procedures applied, and the patient's response to these. Patient charts comprise of Case management, Consent forms, Consultation reports, Contents of patient charts, Core measures, Critical pathways, Flow sheets, Graphic record, History and physical examination form, Kardex records, Laboratory tests record, Medication administration record (MAR), Nurses' notes, Nursing care plans, Other diagnostic reports, Patient education record, Physician's order form, PRN or Unscheduled medication record, Progress notes, and Summary sheet

Safety

Medication errors may result in the failure of completion of a planned action as intended. Medication errors could be prescribing errors, dispensing errors, transcription errors, administration errors, order communication errors, and monitoring errors. Prescribing errors may result from suboptimal decisions with regards to drug therapy, incorrect dosage, prescription of unauthorized drugs or prescription of a drug for a patient with known intolerability or allergy. Dispensing errors may result when a wrong dose or drug is sent or a wrong formulation or dosage is ordered.

Transcription errors result from misinterpreted order regarding a medication or misunderstanding of directions, usage of unapproved abbreviations and illegible handwriting. Administration errors may involve giving an incorrect dosage, missed dose or extra dose, wrong timing of drug administration or incorrect technique or route of administration. Monitoring related errors include improper monitoring, improper assessments of response to drug, and improper patient education regarding the process.

In order to ensure medication safety, some basic principles can be followed. These include the use of CPOE or other technology, use of bar-code for determining status of drug administration and the use of smart pumps to ensure controlled drug administration. Checklists should be used for high alert drugs. Generic and brand names should be used to avoid errors, especially in the case of drugs whose names sound similar. High-alert medication should be restricted during the dispensing process away from the readily available floor stock to ensure that they are not mistakenly taken. Verbal orders should be avoided for high-alert medications. The drug dosing infusion charts and concentrations should be standardized. MTs administering medications should perform double checks before administration.

The patient's current orders of medications should be compared with all the other medications he is taking to avoid errors of duplication, omission, drug interactions and dosage. This kind of medication reconciliation is a five-step procedure beginning with the development of a list of the currently administered medications, along with a list of previously prescribed medications. The two lists need to be compared and clinical decisions are taken depending on the comparison made. The new list is to be communicated to the patient, caregivers, supervisors and other healthcare professionals. Appropriate judgments are to be made with respect to the type of drug, allergies, dosage, therapeutic intent, contraindication and physical preparation of the drug dosage. If a healthcare professional with the responsibility of administering the drug feels it inappropriate to administer the drug, a notification is to be sent to the prescriber immediately along with an explanation for the decision taken.

Medication Administration

There are six rights of medication administration. These are right medication, right dose, right route, right time, right patient and right documentation.

According to the right to right drug, it is crucial to compare the spelling and concentration of the medication prescribed with the drug profile and medication container before administering it.

As per the right to right dosage, it is the responsibility of the medication administrator to double check and confirm the supplied medication matches the ordered dosage and is calculated accurately. The dosage should be confirmed to be appropriate for the patient. He should also pay attention if the patient has any concerns or questions regarding the shape, color or size of the medication.

The medication needs to be administered at the right time. While scheduling the time of drug administration, standardized times, time abbreviations, etc. need to be assessed in order to ensure the maintenance of blood levels, enable maximum absorption of drug and other such factors.

While administering a drug to a patient, the name of the patient on the order or medication card should be cross checked with the name on the bracelet. The patient should also be checked for allergies.

The right route of drug administration is highly crucial in order to ensure the therapeutic efficiency and safety of a drug. The administration of a drug though the IV route delivers it into the blood stream directly. It results in the fastest onset and so, has the highest risk of potential adverse effects. The next fastest absorption occurs upon administration via the intramuscular route depending upon the blood supply availability. However, this route of administration could be painful for the patient. The third fastest route is the subcutaneous route followed by the oral route.

The oral route could be as fast as the intramuscular route depending on the dose form and type of medication, and also on the basis of whether food is present in the stomach of the patient. The oral route is safe for medication administration if a patient is able to swallow and is in a conscious state. The rectal route is to be avoided whenever possible as it causes mucosal tissue irritation and also because its absorption rates are erratic.

Right documentation is another critical requirement during drug administration. The chart and reports should cover the date and time of medication administration, name of drug, route, dosage and the site of the administration of the medication. An incident report regarding an error should mention the date, time of ordering of drug, the name of the drug, route and the dosage. Therapeutic response and adverse effects should be noted.

Different Routes of Medication Administration

The route of drug administration is determined based on the properties of the drug, for instance its solubility and ionization, and by the desired therapeutic action (Harvey, 2008). The major routes of drug administration as described by Harvey (2008) are discussed as follows:

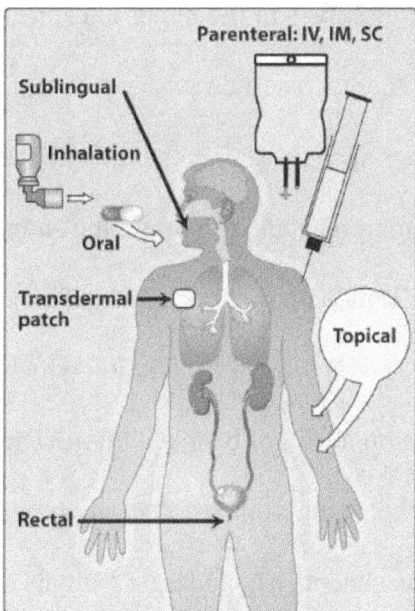

Figure 1: Common routes of administration of medications.

Enteral Route (Oral and Sublingual)

The enteral route of drug administration is the administration of a medication through the mouth, which is the most common, safest, economical and convenient mode. Administration of a medication through the mouth involves swallowing or placing it under the tongue (sublingual). The oral mode of drug administration has many advantages. These can be easily self-administered and pose a low systemic infection risk as compared to the parenteral route, which may have complicated the treatment. Overdose or toxicity resulting from oral administration can be easily reversed through appropriate antidotes such as the use of activated charcoal. However, the pathways associated with oral drug absorption are complicated and the low pH in stomach may also result in drug inactivation. Many kinds of oral drug preparations exist, which include enteric coated preparations and extended release preparations. Enteric coated preparations have an enteric coating which is a chemical envelop that is not affected by the action of enzymes and fluids in the stomach. It dissolves in the upper intestine. This preparation is useful for acid unstable drugs such as omeprazole. Enteric coated drugs are resistant to stomach acid and deliver them in the intestine which is less acidic. Drugs such as aspirin that irritate the stomach can also be coated with a substance that dissolves only in the small intestine to protect the stomach and prevent irritability. Extended release preparations of medications have special ingredients or coatings that control the speed of drug release from the pill. These have a long duration of action which may be required to improve compliance of patients as the medication need not be taken often. These medications maintain their concentrations within an acceptable therapeutic range for a long time, unlike the immediate release forms of drugs whose plasma concentrations generally have larger troughs and peaks. Extended release dosage preparation is suitable for drugs that have short half-lives.

Administration through the sublingual route requires placement of drug under the tongue to facilitate diffusion of the drug into the capillary network and subsequently into the systemic circulation. The advantages of this route are that it facilitates rapid absorption, is easy to administer, has a low incidence of infection, bypasses the gastrointestinal environment which is harsh, and avoids the first-pass metabolism. Another route is the buccal route where the medication is placed between the gum and cheek. This is similar to the sublingual route of medication administration.

Parenteral Route (Intravenous IV, Intramuscular IM, Subcutaneous SC)

The parenteral route of drug administration introduces drugs into the body's systemic circulation against its barrier defenses. This route of administration is suitable for drugs that are poorly absorbed through the gastrointestinal tract and for agents that are unstable in it. It is also useful for treatment of patients who are unconscious and in whom a rapid onset of action is required. Parenteral route of administration has the highest bioavailability and are not subject to the harsh gastrointestinal environment or the first-pass metabolism. It offers most control over the actual dosage of the delivered drug. This mode of administration is irreversible and could induce fear, pain, infections and local tissue damage. The major parenteral routes include intravascular (IV), which could be intra-arterial or intravenous, intramuscular (IM) or subcutaneous (SC). Each of these routes has its own advantages and disadvantages.

The most common parenteral route of medication administration is IV. In case of drugs that cannot be absorbed orally, such as atracurium, a neuromuscular blocker, there is often no choice other than IV. This mode of drug delivery enables a rapid effect and offers the maximum degree of control over the drug's circulating levels. When the drug is injected as bolus, the entire drug is immediately delivered into the systemic circulation. Through IV infusion, the same dose can be administered over a longer time because of which the peak in plasma concentration decreases and the drug is present in the circulation over a longer period of time. IV injection is suitable while administering medications that cause irritation through other routes as the blood dilutes them rapidly. However, injected drugs cannot be recalled using strategies such as activated charcoal unlike those that are administered via the gastrointestinal tract.

Another disadvantage of IV injection is that it may inadvertently introduce infectious agents such as bacteria through contamination, and it may also precipitate the constituents of blood. It may also induce hemolysis and result in other adverse effects due to a very rapid delivery of high drug concentrations into the tissues and plasma. Patients administered through this route need to be monitored carefully for adverse drug reactions so that careful control of the rate of infusion can be carried out.

The IM route of drug administration involves the use of an aqueous solution that facilitates rapid absorption. Specialized depot preparations can be used when slow absorption is required. Depot preparations use a nonaqueous vehicle containing a suspension of the drug. The drug precipitates at injection site in the muscle as the vehicle diffuses out. The drug slowly dissolves and a sustained dosage is provided for an extended time period. Some drugs administered through this mode include medroxyprogesterone (depot) and haloperidol (sustained-release).

Subcutaneous route of medication administration is slightly slower than the IV route and absorption is through diffusion. It minimizes the risk of thrombosis and hemolysis that has a greater frequency of occurrence when the route of administration is IV injection. The SC route is not used for drugs that result in tissue irritation, because it may result in necrosis and pain. An example is that of epinephrine, minute amounts of which are combined with a subcutaneously administered drug to confine its area of action. Other examples include etonogestrel.

Inhalation and Intrathecal/Intraventricular Route

Drugs can also be administered through inhalation, both nasal and oral. This route enables rapid drug delivery across mucous membranes of pulmonary epithelium and the respiratory tract, which have a large surface area. The effect of this route is as rapid as IV injection and it is used for gaseous drugs such as certain anesthetics that can be dispersed using an aerosol.

Administration through oral inhalation is highly effective for patients having respiratory disorders such as asthma as the drug is directly delivered to the site of action. This route minimizes side effects. Some of the drugs that are administered via this route include albuterol, a bronchodilator and fluticasone, a corticosteroid.

The nasal inhalation route of administration involves delivery via the nose using nasal sprays. Nasal decongestants like oxymetazoline are administered through this route. Another route is the intrathecal/intraventricular route. This route is used to deliver drugs directly into the cerebrospinal fluid because the blood-brain barrier delays drug absorption into the central nervous system.

Topical, Transdermal and Rectal Routes

Some drugs are applied topically for a local effect. Examples include clotrimazole, a cream that is applied directly on the skin for treating dermatophytosis. The transdermal route of administration is used when systemic effects are desired by applying drugs on the skin, usually using a transdermal patch. This route is used when a sustained delivery of drugs is required. For instance, scopolamine, an antiemetic is administered using a transdermal patch. The rectal route of administration of medication is employed to prevent destruction of drugs by intestinal enzymes or due to fluids or low pH in the stomach. It also minimizes the liver biotransformation of drugs. This route is also suitable if a drug causes vomiting through oral ingestion, if a patient is already in the condition of vomiting, or if he is not conscious for oral administration. It is commonly used for the administration of antiemetics.

Drugs Affecting Various Systems of the Human Body

Medications target different systems of the human body and are classified accordingly. Some important drug categories that act on the various systems are discussed here (Rosenfeld and Loose, 2014; Aehlert and Vroman, 2011):

Drugs Affecting the Cardiovascular System

Drugs that are used for the treatment of congestive heart failure (CHF) include angiotensin-converting enzyme (ACE) inhibitors such as Captopril and Enalapril, and angiotensin receptor blockers (ARBs) such as Valsartan. Other drugs used for the treatment of CHF are cardiac glycosides and inotropic agents such as milrinone. Diuretics and vasodilators are also used. Antiarrhythmic drugs used for treatment of Arrhythmias include Quinidine and Procainamide. Antianginal agents include nitrates and nitirites, β-Adrenoceptor antagonists and Calcium channel-blocking agents (CCB) such as Nifedipine. Antihypertensive drugs include β-Adrenoceptor antagonists such as Propranolol and α-Adrenoceptor antagonists such as Labetalol. Renin inhibitors such as Aliskiren, antihypertensive agents such as hydralazine, and specialized vasodilators such as Ambrisentan are some of the other drugs that affect the cardiovascular system.

Drugs Affecting the Urinary System

Some of the drugs that affect the urinary system include diuretics such as Thiazide diuretics, Thiazide-like drugs such as chlorthalidone and loop diuretics such as furosemide. Carbonic anhydrase inhibitors used for treatment of glaucoma are also used for enhancing the renal secretion of cysteine and uric acid. Agents that influence the excretion of water include osmotic agents like mannitol and urea. Nondiuretic inhibitors, Uricosuric agents and other agents such as Allopurinol are also employed in treatment of disorders related to the urinary system.

Drugs Affecting the Respiratory System

Drugs affecting the respiratory system include decongestants, antitussives, expectorants, antihistamines, and mucolytics. Antitussives used for controlling nonproductive cough include codeine, benzonatate and Dextromethorphan. Other drugs that affect the respiratory system include topical nasal decongestants such as Ephedrine, oral decongestants, topical nasal steroids such as Flunisolide, antihistamines such as Diphenhydramine, expectorants such as Guaifenesin and mucolytics such as acetylcysteine.

Drugs Affecting the Digestive System, Vitamins, and Minerals

Drugs affecting the digestive system include those that are used for peptic ulcers and those that are used to modulate gastroentric functions. Anti-ulcer drugs include antacids, drugs such as muscarinic receptor antagonists, H2 receptor antagonists, proton pump inhibitors that inhibit secretion of gastric acid, mucosal protective drugs and antimicrobial drugs. Common antacids include Aluminium hydroxide and Magnesium trisilicate. Muscarinic receptor antagonists include Atropine and Telenzepine. H2 receptor antagonists include Ranitidine, proton pump inhibitors include Omeprazole. Mucosal protective drugs include Misoprostol and Marzulene. Antimicrobial drugs include Tetracycline and Amoxicillin. Modulator drugs influencing gastroenteric functions include antiemetic (Diphenhydramine, Scopolamine, etc.) and prokinetic drugs (Metoclopramide, Domperidone, etc.), laxatives (Phenolphthalein, Magnesium sulfate, etc.) and diarrhea treating drugs (Diphenoxylate, Tannalbin, etc.).

Drugs Affecting the Central Nervous System (CNS)

Drugs affecting the CNS include depressants such as sedatives and hypnotics, which include Barbiturates, Benzodiazepines, etc. Sedative-hypnotic drugs include flurazepam, which is long acting, and estazolam, which is short acting. Anxiolytic (anxiety relieving) drugs include alprazolam, lorazepam, diazepam and chloridiazepoxide.

Drugs Affecting the Musculoskeletal System

These include uricosuric drugs such as colchicine, indomethacin (a non-steroidal antiinflammatry drug, and allopurinol). Colchicine is used for relieving the symptoms of gout. It is an alkaloid that suppresses the initial immune reaction responsible for pain.

Drugs Affecting the Endocrine System

Drugs affecting the pituitary gland include octreotide, somatrem and sermorelin for the anterior pituitary gland and vasopressin and desmopressin for the posterior pituitary gland. Drugs affecting the thyroid and parathyroid are calciferol, plicamycin, liotrix and levothyroxine. In addition, certain steroids and corticosteroids influence the adrenal cortex. These include hydrocortisone, dexamethasone, hydrocortisone sodium succinate and fludrocortisone.

Antibiotics and Other Anti-Infective Agents

These include aerosolized anti-infective agents such as Pentamidine isethionate, Ribavirin, and Zanamivir; aerosolized antibiotics, non-aerosolized anti-infective agents such as cell wall affecting agents like Penicillins, Bacitracin, Vancomycin, protein synthesis inhibiting agents like Chloramphenicol, Streptomycin, Kanamycin, Lincomycin, Gentamicin, and Aminoglycosides and nucleic acid synthesis inhibiting agents like Mitomycin, Rifampicin and Actinomycin.

Antibiotics are classified as bactericidal (Cephalosporins, Streptomycin, Cycloserine, Penicillins, Polymyxins, Kanamycin) and bacteriostatic (Tetracyclines, Chloramphenicol, Erythromycin). They are also classified alternatively as broad spectrum (Chloramphenicol, Cephalosporins, Ampicillin, Kanamycin) and narrow spectrum (Erythromycin, Polymyxin B, Penicillin).

Synthetic (nonantibiotic) anti-infective agents include Sulfonamides (Sulfamethoxazole, Sulfisoxazole, Sulfamethizole, Sulfacytine), Trimethoprim-Sulfamethoxazole and Nitrofurantoin. Antifungal agents include Nystatin, Amphotericin B and Griseofulvin. Antituberculosis agents include Streptomycin, Pyrazinamide, Rifampin, Isoniazid and Ethambutol. Antiviral agents include Acyclovir, Didanosine, Ganciclovir, Idoxuridine, Rimantadine and Vidarabine.

Drugs Affecting the Eye and Ear

Drugs applied to the eye may have many purposes which include treatment of a medical condition, prevention of eye infection and for the enhancement of eye examination. Some of the drugs affecting the eye include antiglaucoma agents, cycloplegic and mydriatic agents, topical anesthetic agents, anti-infective agents, anti-inflammatory agents, and other ophthalmic preparations. Anti-glaucoma agents used to treat glaucoma include beta blockers such as betaxolol and timolol, carbonic anhydrase inhibitors such as acetazolamide, prostaglandin analogs such as latanoprost, sympathomimetics such as brimonidine and other agents such as pilocarpine. Cycloplegic and mydriatic agents are administered to dilate the pupil and to treat inflammation and pain.

Examples of these agents include cyclopentolate hydrochloride, epinephrine, homatropine ophthalmic solution, and atropine ophthalmic solution. Topical anesthetic agents are used as local anesthetics for pain reduction. These include proparacaine HCL and tetracocaine HCL. Other preparations used for ophthalmic administration include lubricants and artificial tears. Drugs affecting the ear include anti-inflammatory agents, antibiotics and wax buildup suppressing agents. Topical otic preparatons such as drops usually contain antibiotics.

Conclusion

This study guide introduced the healthcare profession of a medication technician and discussed his/her functions and responsibilities. It also discussed the various principles of drug administration, the importance of accurate medical history and how medication errors can be avoided. Various routes of drug administration have also been summarized with examples. The study guides also lists out important categories of drugs affecting important systems of the human body.

References

Aehlert, B., & Vroman, R. (2011). *Paramedic Practice Today: Above and Beyond*. Massachusetts: Jones & Bartlett Publishers.

Clayton, B. D. (2012). *Basic Pharmacology for Nurses16: Basic Pharmacology for Nurses*. Missouri: Elsevier Health Sciences.

Durgin, J. M., & Hanan, Z. I. (2004). *Thomson Delmar Learning's Pharmacy Practice for Technicians*. New York: Cengage Learning.

FitzGerald, R. J. (2009). Medication errors: the importance of an accurate drug history. *British Journal of Clinical Pharmacology, 67*(6), 671-675.

Flynn, E. A. (n.d.). *A brief history of medication errors*. Retrieved from http://www.medaccuracy.com/Papers%20and%20Publications/A%20Brief%20History%20 of%20Medication%20Errors.pdf.

French, L., & Fordney, M. (2012). *Administrative Medical Assisting*. New York: Cengage Learning.

Harvey, R. (2008). *Lippincott's Illustrated Review: Pharmacology*. Pennsylvania: Lippincott Williams & Wilkins.

Maryland Board of Nursing. (2008, February 27). *Medicine Aides versus Medication Technicians - What's the Difference*. Retrieved from http://www.mbon.org/main.php?v=norm&c=medtech/medaide_vs_medtech.html.

Whitenton, L., & Walker, M. (2013). *MACE Exam Cram: Medication Aide Certification Exam*. Pearson Certification.

Practice Questions. Section One

1. Which of the following is the responsibility of the medication aide?
   a. Diagnosing patients
   b. Prescribing medications
   c. Administering and distributing medication to patients
   d. Titrating medications

2. The main role of a medication technician should be:
   a. Administer daily medications to patients
   b. Prescribe medications to patients
   c. Fill prescriptions for patients
   d. None of the above

3. Which of the following are roles of the medication technician?
   a. Check vital signs
   b. Administer medication to patients
   c. Observe the patient
   d. All of the above

4. Which of the following should a medication technician never do?
   a. Administer the first dose of a new medication
   b. Watch the patient for side effects
   c. Follow medication guidelines
   d. All of the above

5. What is a thermometer used for?
   a. Assessing the pulse of a patient
   b. Measuring blood pressure of a patient
   c. Measuring body temperature
   d. Assessing the responsiveness of a patient

6. An oral thermometer produces a reading of 101 degrees Fahrenheit. This patient is:
   a. Febrile
   b. Afebrile
   c. Normal
   d. None of the above

7. A medication tech ought to report:
   a. Changes in a patient's physical state
   b. Changes in a patient's mental state
   c. Changes in a patient's emotional state
   d. All of the above

8. A fever that remains constant is:
   a. Remittent
   b. Afebrile
   c. Continuous
   d. Intermittent

9. Which of the following should a medication technician be aware of?
   a. Special instructions on giving medications
   b. Procedures and protocol
   c. Side effects of the medication
   d. All of the above

10. Who should not have their temperatures taken orally?
    a. Elderly patients
    b. Patients receiving oxygen
    c. Teenage patients
    d. Patients with broken ribs

11. Which patients should not have temperatures taken rectally?
    a. Patients with NG tubes
    b. Patients with diarrhea
    c. Infants
    d. Patients who smoke

12. A nurse has asked you to administer medication to a patient with an NG tube. You should:
    a. Respectfully explain that you cannot administer medications via NG tubes
    b. Give the medications to the patient
    c. Tell her that you administered the dose, but don't
    d. None of the above

13. How should a pulse be taken?
    a. With the first two or three fingers for about thirty seconds
    b. With the third and fourth finger on the femoral artery
    c. With the thumb on the jugular
    d. With the thumb on the brachial artery

14. Which of the following counts as a respiration?
    a. An inhalation
    b. An inhalation and an exhalation
    c. An exhalation

d. A cough

15. The apical pulse is taken:
    a. With the first and second finger
    b. Over the apex of the heart with the palm of the hand
    c. Over the apex of the heart with a stethoscope
    d. None of the above

16. Vital signs reflect:
    a. Status of the patient
    b. The functions of the body processes necessary for life
    c. The Effects of medications on the patient
    d. All of the above

17. The apical pulse is especially useful in:
    a. Infants or small children
    b. In the elderly
    c. In patients with brittle bones
    d. In patients going into fibrillation

18. When taking a pulse you should feel:
    a. On the radial artery which is located at the chest.
    b. On the brachial artery on the back side of the arm
    c. On the temporal artery located on the forehead
    d. On the radial artery located on the same side as the patient's thumb

19. Tachypnea is characterized by:
    a. A rate of breathing greater than 40 breaths per minute
    b. A rate of breathing less than 10 breaths per minute
    c. A rate of breathing greater than 20 breaths per minute
    d. A rate of breathing less than 5 breaths per minute

20. A patient has a fever that has been fluctuating all day. However, the fever never returns to a baseline or a normal temperature. This is considered:
    a. Continuous fever
    b. Intermittent fever
    c. Remittent fever
    d. Afebrile fever

21. Apnea occurs when:
    a. The patient permanently stops breathing
    b. The patient temporarily has complete absence of breath
    c. The patient is in hysteria
    d. The patient is breathing normally

22. Bradypnea:
    a. Occurs when a patient hyperventilates
    b. Has a breathing rate of greater than 40 breaths per minute
    c. Is normal during a sleeping state
    d. Is never normal

23. Depth of respiration refers to:
    a. Number of breaths per minutes
    b. Amount of air inspired and expired
    c. Number of heartbeats per minute
    d. Amount of blood pumped through the heart per minute

24. Hypoventilation refers to a time when:
    a. Reduced air enters the lungs
    b. Increased air enters the lungs
    c. Normal amounts of air enters the lungs
    d. No air enters the lungs

25. A patient has an IV and is getting medications through the IV drip. The nurse is busy, but it is time to replace the medication bag. You should:
    a. Help out by changing the IV and setting the pump
    b. Leave everything alone
    c. Notify the nurse that something needs to be done
    d. None of the above

26. Hypoventilation results in:
    a. Excess oxygen in the blood and decreased carbon dioxide in the blood
    b. Excess nitrogen in the blood and decreased carbon dioxide
    c. Decreased nitrogen in the blood and increased oxygen in the blood
    d. Decreased oxygen in the blood and increased carbon dioxide

27. Anthropometric measurements refers to:
    a. Measurements of the heart and lungs
    b. Comparative measurements of the body
    c. Comparative measurements of lung function
    d. All of the above

28. Most accidents occur because:
    a. The patient does not cooperate
    b. Rules are overlooked or ignored
    c. Healthcare professionals don't care
    d. None of the above

29. Which of the following is an example of a hazard in the healthcare setting?
    a. Electrical hazards
    b. Biological hazards

c. Chemical hazards
d. All of the above

30. A coworker has noticed a stripped cord connected to a bed. This is an example of:
    a. Electrical hazards
    b. Biological hazards
    c. Chemical hazards
    d. Neurological hazards

31. Someone has left out some strong cleaning supplies. This is an example of:
    a. Electrical hazards
    b. Biological hazards
    c. Chemical hazards
    d. Neurological hazards

32. Someone has left out an uncapped, used sharp. This is an example of:
    a. Electrical hazards
    b. Biological hazards
    c. Chemical hazards
    d. Neurological hazards

33. Which of the following is not an anthropometric measurement?
    a. Lucidity
    b. Weight
    c. Height
    d. Head circumference

34. A coworker has cut himself badly on a jagged piece of metal. You should:
    a. Have the coworker lie down
    b. Pour disinfectant on the wound
    c. Apply pressure and elevate the wound
    d. Perform CPR

35. A patient is on the floor with cold/clammy skin, blank expression, and shallow breathing. This patient possibly is suffering from:
    a. Shock
    b. Stroke
    c. Heart attack
    d. Sun poisoning

36. CPR stands for:
    a. Cardio-Palpitative Resuscitation
    b. Carotid-Pulmonary Recognizance
    c. Cardio-Pulmonary Resuscitation
    d. Carotid-Palliative Recognizance

37. An influenza virus is an example of:
    a. An agent
    b. A portal of exit
    c. A mode of transmission
    d. A portal of entry

38. Which of the following is not an example of a portal of entry?
    a. A scratch on the hand
    b. Intact skin
    c. A mucous membrane
    d. Respiratory tract

39. Which of the following is not an example of a mode of transmission?
    a. Air borne
    b. handwashing
    c. Contact
    d. Body Fluid

40. Which of the following means "the destruction of pathogenic microorganisms after they leave the body"?
    a. Vector transmission
    b. Asymmetry
    c. Medical Asepsis
    d. Organ Sepsis

41. When disinfecting items you should:
    a. Use chemicals on every item to be disinfected
    b. Put everything into a cleaning oven
    c. Wipe everything down with water
    d. Use chemicals only on inanimate objects

42. Which item would not be eligible to be cleaned with boiling water?
    a. An oral thermometer
    b. A pair of utility scissors
    c. A reflex hammer
    d. A mug

43. Surgical instruments are placed in an autoclave. This is an example of:
    a. Dry heat sterilization
    b. Chemical sterilization
    c. Steam sterilization
    d. Gas sterilization

44. A wheelchair is placed in a chamber for sterilization. This is most likely an example of:
    a. Dry heat sterilization
    b. Chemical sterilization

c. Steam sterilization

d. Gas sterilization

45. The most important way of fighting infection is:
    a. Dry heat sterilization
    b. Hand washing
    c. Cleaning things with bleach
    d. All of the above

46. You must wear a face shield for performing a procedure. This is an example of:
    a. Isolation
    b. Medical asepsis
    c. Barrier protection
    d. Contact asepsis

47. Standard precautions include which of the following?
    a. Wearing gloves
    b. Wearing face shields when necessary
    c. Disposing of sharps without recapping
    d. All of the above

48. In order to prevent airborne diseases from spreading you should use:
    a. Universal precautions
    b. Contact precautions
    c. Airborne precautions
    d. All of the above

49. You catch a cold after you drink with the same cup your daughter used. This is an example of:
    a. Airborne contamination
    b. Indirect contact transmission
    c. Direct contact transmission
    d. Vector transmission

50. A patient has a cold. This could be transmitted through:
    a. Airborne
    b. Contact
    c. Body Fluid
    d. All of the above

51. A child develops a rash after playing closely with another child. This could be an example of:
    a. Direct contact transmission
    b. Airborne transmission
    c. Vector transmission
    d. Indirect contact transmission

52. A virus is an example of a:
   a. Susceptible host
   b. An agent
   c. A vector
   d. Portal of exit

53. Standard precautions are aimed at:
   a. Preventing the spread of infectious agents as they exit the reservoir
   b. Preventing the spread of infectious as they enter the susceptible host
   c. Preventing the spread of infectious agents as they travel through the air
   d. None of the above

54. When a person appears to be in shock you should:
   a. Have the person sit up and elevate the arms
   b. Have the person stand up and elevate the arms
   c. Have the person lay down and elevate the feet
   d. None of the above

55. When should you wash your hands?
   a. Before and after speaking with the patient
   b. Before and after entering a room
   c. After eating and using the bathroom
   d. After leaving the hospital

56. To avoid chemical hazards you should always:
   a. Store chemicals with non-hazardous materials
   b. Pour chemicals into clear bottles
   c. Label all chemicals with the MSDS
   d. All of the above

57. In order to avoid biological hazards you should:
   a. Incinerate any non-cleanable materials
   b. Sterilize any materials that can be sterilized
   c. Wash hands before and after each procedure
   d. All of the above

58. To avoid electrical hazards you should:
   a. Never use extension cords
   b. Replace any cords that are bare or have the wire showing
   c. Unplug electrical equipment before servicing
   d. All of the above

59. When an accident occurs you should:
   a. Attempt to clean up the mess before anyone notices
   b. Talk about it with a co-worker
   c. Report it to a supervisor

d. Leave it for someone else

60. Cheyne-Stokes refers to:
    a. Regular pattern of irregular breathing
    b. Irregular pattern of regular breathing
    c. Regular pattern of regular breathing
    d. Irregular pattern of irregular breathing

61. Orthopnea refers to:
    a. Trouble breathing because of problems with the rib bones
    b. Regular breathing in an inverted position
    c. Difficulty breathing when not upright
    d. Difficulty breathing when upright

62. Apnea refers to:
    a. A period of increased breathing, then returning to normal
    b. A period of no breath
    c. A period of decreased breath depth
    d. None of the above

63. When using a rectal thermometer:
    a. All patients are eligible for rectal thermometers
    b. Only babies should have rectal temperatures taken
    c. Only elderly patients should have rectal temperatures taken
    d. Patients with heart disease should not have rectal temperatures taken

64. If a patient has just been drinking or smoking you should:
    a. Take temperature orally anyway
    b. Wait thirty minutes and then take his/her temperature
    c. Wait ten minutes and then take temperature rectally
    d. None of the above

65. A patient is described as afebrile. This patient is:
    a. Having heart trouble
    b. Having breathing trouble
    c. Has a normal body temperature
    d. Has fertility problems

66. A patient has an axillary temperature of 98 degrees Fahrenheit. This patient:
    a. Has a normal body temperature
    b. Has a low body temperature
    c. Has a high body temperature
    d. Should be tested with an oral thermometer

67. Which of the following is not a place to take a temperature?
    a. Axillary area
    b. Rectal area
    c. Antecubital area
    d. Eye

68. Why is it important to get an accurate medication history?
    a. To find out how the patient reacted to medications in the past
    b. So you can tell the nurse
    c. To write in the chart
    d. All of the above

69. Medication history includes which of the following?
    a. Current medications
    b. Current and past health history
    c. Supplements
    d. All of the above

70. Which of the following should be reported with the medication history?
    a. Vitamins and minerals
    b. Previous reactions to medications
    c. Herbal supplements
    d. All of the above

71. The patient has brought medications with him. The medication tech should:
    a. Examine the medication for dosage and frequency
    b. Tell the nurse that the patient brought the meds
    c. Record the medications brought in the 'patient's own medication' section.
    d. All of the above

72. A nurse has asked you to administer medication to a patient with an NG tube. You should:
    a. Respectfully explain that you cannot administer medications via NG tubes
    b. Give the medications to the patient
    c. Tell her that you administered the dose, but don't
    d. None of the above

73. A patient seems suddenly lethargic after being given medications. This could be a sign of:
    a. Sleepiness
    b. Apathy
    c. Adverse reaction

d. Anger

74. You have given a patient a medication and her tongue starts to swell. This is an example of:
    a. Emotional reaction
    b. Physical reaction
    c. Psychological reaction
    d. None of the above

75. A patient who was fairly happy is suddenly depressed on the third day after starting a medication. This is an example of:
    a. Emotional reaction
    b. Physical reaction
    c. The reaction is fake
    d. None of the above

76. A patient is given a medication and starts seeing things (visual hallucination). This is an example of:
    a. The reaction is fake
    b. Physical reaction
    c. Psychological reaction
    d. None of the above

77. A patient develops a rash after taking medication. You should:
    a. Notify the nurse
    b. Record it in the chart
    c. Observe the patient for further reaction
    d. All of the above

78. A patient has an insulin pump and asks you to help program it. You should:
    a. Explain to the patient that you can find help
    b. Help program the pump
    c. Leave the room
    d. Say no and walk away

79. A patient has an IV and is getting medications through the IV drip. The nurse is busy, but it is time to replace the medication bag. You should:
    a. Help out by changing the IV and setting the pump
    b. Leave everything alone
    c. Notify the nurse that something needs to be done

d. None of the above

80. Which of the following should a medication technician be aware of?
    a. Special instructions on giving medications
    b. Procedures and protocol
    c. Side effects of the medication
    d. All of the above

81. A medication tech ought to report:
    a. Changes in a patient's physical state
    b. Changes in a patient's mental state
    c. Changes in a patient's emotional state
    d. All of the above

82. Which of the following statements is true?
    a. Supplements can complement or inhibit prescription medications
    b. Most patients do not record the dosage of their supplements
    c. Supplements can affect clotting
    d. All of the above

83. The medication aide can also admit patients.
    a. True
    b. False

84. The main role of a medication technician should be:
    a. Administer daily medications to patients
    b. Prescribe medications to patients
    c. Fill prescriptions for patients
    d. None of the above

85. Which of the following is true?
    a. A medication technician should trust the nurse/doctor and give medications without asking questions
    b. A medication technician only has to measure out prescribed medications
    c. A medication technician should cross check medications and dosage in order to prevent errors
    d. All above are true

86. Medication history could be obtained through:
    a. Family members

b. Patient

c. Patient's chart

d. All of the above

87. Which of the following should be reported with the medication history?

a. Vitamins and minerals

b. Previous reactions to medications

c. Herbal supplements

d. All of the above

88. Not obtaining a medication history could lead to serious errors.

a. True

b. False

89. A nurse has asked you to administer medication to a patient with an NG tube. You should:

a. Respectfully explain that you cannot administer medications via NG tubes

b. Give the medications to the patient

c. Tell her that you administered the dose, but don't

d. None of the above

90. The right to refuse a medication is one of the patient's rights.

A. True

B. False

91. To measure an apical pulse, one needs a stethoscope.

a. True

b. False

92. When taking a pulse you should:

a. Assume the number of respiration is the same as the pulse

b. Record how many pulse per day

c. Record how many pulse per hour

d. Record how many pulse per minute

93. Bradypnea is characterized by:

a. A rate of breathing greater than 40 breaths per minute

b. A rate of breathing less than 10 breaths per minute

c. A rate of breathing greater than 100 breaths per minute

d. A rate of breathing less than 50 breaths per minute

94. When obtaining a blood pressure, cuffs that are too short or narrow may give falsely high readings

a. True

b. False

95. Blood pressure is recorded in:
    a. Cm(centimeters)
    b. mmhg (millimeter mercury)
    c. Dl (Decilitres)
    d. Km (Kilo meters)

96. Bradypnea:
    a. Occurs when a patient hyperventilates
    b. Has a breathing rate of greater than 40 breaths per minute
    c. Is normal during a sleeping state
    d. Is never normal

97. Depth of respiration refers to:
    a. Number of breaths per minutes
    b. Amount of air inspired and expired
    c. Number of heartbeats per minute
    d. Amount of blood pumped through the heart per minute

98. Hypoventilation refers to a time when:
    a. Reduced air enters the lungs
    b. Increased air enters the lungs
    c. Normal amounts of air enters the lungs
    d. No air enters the lungs

99. A patient has a wound that is due changing. The nurse is busy, but it is time to replace the change the wound. You should:
    a. Help out by changing the wound
    b. Leave everything alone
    c. Notify the nurse that something needs to be done
    d. None of the above

100.   Hypoventilation results in:
    a. Excess oxygen in the blood and decreased carbon dioxide in the blood
    b. Excess nitrogen in the blood and decreased carbon dioxide
    c. Decreased nitrogen in the blood and increased oxygen in the blood
    d. Decreased oxygen in the blood and increased carbon dioxide

Section Two Medication Aide Practice Questions

1. What is a common problem in medical histories?
   a. Failure to report medications
   b. Failure to report supplements
   c. Failure to explore hypersensitivities
   d. All of the above

2. Which of the following should an MT do before administering medications?
   a. Talk to the patient and answer questions
   b. Ask the patient to go to the bathroom.
   c. Check the IV
   d. Check the patient's temperature

3. Which of the following is essential to good patient care?
   a. Handwashing
   b. Privacy
   c. Communication
   d. All of the above

4. When should the MT wash his/her hands?
   a. Before administering meds only
   b. After administering meds only
   c. Before and after administering meds
   d. In the morning when he/she showers

5. One of the main causes of medication errors is:
   a. Nurses being too busy to be careful
   b. Untrained medical staff
   c. Inability of patients to accurately report drug history
   d. All of the above

6. Which of the following should the medication technician be familiar with?
   a. Reasons for prescribed medication
   b. Expected adverse reactions
   c. The 5 rights of medication administration
   d. All of the above

7. Which of the following would be found in the patient's chart?
   a. Flow sheets
   b. Vital signs
   c. Consent forms
   d. All of the above

8. Where would you find the doctor's orders?
   a. The nurse's station

b. The chart

c. The whiteboard

d. Medical record's department

9. In order to prevent medication errors:
    a. Trust the patient's memory about medications
    b. Administer drug orders received verbally
    c. Bar codes, checklists, and smart pumps should be used
    d. All of the above

10. As a technician you should:
    a. Follow orders without question
    b. Check the medications prescribed for accuracy
    c. Let the nurse administer medications
    d. Adjust dosage as you see fit

11. Which "right" says that spelling and concentration of medication should be checked?
    a. Right dose
    b. Right drug
    c. Right route
    d. Right time

12. Which "right" requires you to check dosage?
    a. Right dose
    b. Right drug
    c. Right time
    d. Right route

13. Which "right" determines how the drug enters the patient's body?
    a. Right patient
    b. Right documentation
    c. Right route
    d. Right time

14. Which route has the fastest drug absorption rate?
    a. Sublingual
    b. Subdermal
    c. IV
    d. Oral

15. Which route should be avoided if possible?
    a. Sublingual
    b. Rectal
    c. Intramuscular
    d. Oral

16. What medication property is not considered when choosing a route for a drug?
    a. Solubility
    b. Desired therapeutic action
    c. Nurses' comfortability
    d. Ionization properties

17. Which of the following is not a word for taking medication by mouth?
    a. Oral
    b. Sublingual
    c. Enteral
    d. Subdermal

18. In order to protect certain medications from stomach acid, the medications may be:
    a. Taken rectally
    b. Coated with a protective capsule
    c. Crushed and mixed with applesauce
    d. Taken with milk

19. Which of the following describes a route that has rapid absorption, is easy to administer, and bypasses the GI tract?
    a. Oral
    b. Sublingual
    c. IV
    d. Intramuscular

20. Which of the following is the same as "parental" route?
    a. Intravenous
    b. Intramuscular
    c. Subcutaneous
    d. All of the above

21. Which of the following is a disadvantage of IV drug administration?
    a. The drug cannot be neutralized/recalled
    b. The drug can be delivered over a period of time
    c. The drug is delivered directly into the circulatory system
    d. There is no disadvantage

22. Which of the following is a risk of the IV route?
    a. The results are close to immediate
    b. There is a great deal of control
    c. Giving the IV could bring pain and even infection
    d. The rate of delivery can be controlled

23. A patient is to receive a drug parentally. This medication can cause tissue irritation. Which way would this medication definitely not be administered?
    a. Through IV

b. Subcutaneously

c. Inhalation

d. It can be given all of these ways

24. Which route is as effective as IV administration and is used for gaseous medications?

    a. Subcutaneous

    b. Inhalation

    c. Sublingual

    d. Intramuscular

25. Which of the following statements is true?

    a. All drugs affect the body equally

    b. All drugs affect only one system

    c. Drugs are classified based on the system that they affect

    d. Drugs usually target the whole body

26. A drug is considered a decongestant. The medication most likely affects:

    a. Urinary tract

    b. Neurology

    c. The kidneys

    d. The respiratory tract

27. A medication is used to stop chest pains. This medication most likely affects:

    a. The heart

    b. The mind

    c. The soul

    d. None of the above

28. A medication is specified for use on peptic ulcers. This medication affects:

    a. The heart

    b. The digestive tract

    c. The respiratory tract

    d. The gallbladder

29. A medication that reduces the amount of fluid in various parts of the body is called:

    a. Nitroglycerine

    b. Cortisols

    c. Diuretic

    d. Beta inhibitors

30. Sedative medications affect:

    a. Nervous system

    b. Respiratory system

    c. Digestive system

    d. Urinary tract

31. Drugs that affect the thyroid or the pituitary glands affect the:
    a. Nervous system
    b. Endocrine system
    c. Circulatory system
    d. Nephrological system

32. A patch that delivers medication over a period of time delivers the medication:
    a. Transdermally
    b. Via inhaler
    c. Orally
    d. Subcutaneously

33. A patient is unconscious. Which way should medication not be administered to this patient?
    a. Intravenously
    b. Rectally
    c. Orally
    d. Subdermally

34. Which of the following needs to be considered when deciding whether or not a patient should be given medication orally?
    a. Ability to swallow
    b. Whether or not the medication can withstand the digestive tract
    c. Consciousness of the patient
    d. All of the above

35. You enter a patient's room. Before giving the patient medication you should:
    a. Wash your hands
    b. Check the patient's name
    c. Check the drug dosage
    d. All of the above

36. You notice that a medication has been ordered for a patient. When you took the patient's medical history you noted that the patient had a bad reaction to this medication. You should:
    a. Give the patient the medication anyway
    b. Skip the dose
    c. Notify the nurse and the prescriber
    d. Dilute the medication

37. You notice that a medication that interacts with another medication has been prescribed. You notified the proper people. You should also:
    a. Wash your hands
    b. Give the medication anyway
    c. Note it in the chart
    d. Talk to the patient

38. A patient's friend is curious about the patient's medication. You should:
    a. Tell the friend about the medical problems of the patient
    b. Let the friend administer the medication
    c. Tell the friend to mind her own business
    d. Explain politely that you cannot talk about the patient's medical condition

39. Which of the following is essential to good patient care?
    a. Handwashing
    b. Privacy
    c. Communication
    d. All of the above

40. Handwashing is the single most effective way to prevent the spread of infection.
    a.   True
    b.   False

41. Why are vital signs taken on admission?
    a.   To obtain the baseline health information on the patient
    b.   To fulfill the admission process
    c.   To make the patient feel welcome.

42. If a patient refuses medication, what should the MT do?
    a. Document the refusal
    b. Let the nurse know
    c. A &B
    d. Force the patient to take medication

43. Which of the following would be found in the patient's chart?
    a. Flow sheets
    b. Vital signs
    c. Consent forms
    d. All of the above

44. Where would you find the doctor's orders?
    a. The nurse's station
    b. The patient's bracelet
    c. The chart
    d. Medical record's department

45. You wake up one morning feeling ill. You know that the illness could make a patient ill. You should:
    a. Go to work anyway
    b. Take medication and wait to see how you feel
    c. Call in sick to work
    d. Diagnose yourself

46. A Medication Technician is required to take continuing education courses to renew certification.
    a. True
    b. False

47. You find that a patient was previously hypersensitive to a medication. You should:
    a. Note it
    b. Ask more questions about the reaction
    c. Alert the nurse/physician
    d. All of the above

48. In order to prevent medication errors:
    a. Bar codes should be used to track medications
    b. You should let the patient administer his/her own meds
    c. Only the doctor should give medication
    d. All of the above

49. Which of the following is essential to being a successful MT?
    a. Confidentiality
    b. Good hygiene
    c. Respect for the patient
    d. All of the above

50. Which of the following BPs is abnormal?
    a. 160/100mmhg
    b. 85/40mmhg
    c. 80/50mmhg
    d. All of the above

51. Why is oral thermometers not used in a mental health patient?
    a. They could bite on it and hurt themselves
    b. Oral thermometers could be used on them
    c. They have no oral temperature

52. Why is rectal thermometer not used in patients who have diarrhea?
    a. They have no rectal temperature
    b. The thermometer insertion could stimulate the nerves and continue the diarrhea
    c. They can be used on them

53. Sublingual medications are:
    a. Placed under the tongue
    b. Swallowed
    c. Chewed before swallowing
    d. Drunk with juice

54. Uricosuric agents and other agents such as Allopurinol are also employed in treatment of disorders related to the _____.

a. Digestive system
b. Urinary system
c. cardiovascular system
d. musculoskeletal system

55. Drugs affecting the pituitary gland include:
    a. Octreotide
    b. Somatrem
    c. Sermorelin
    d. All of the above

56. . Some of the drugs affecting the eye include:
    a.   Antiglaucoma agents
    b.   Cycloplegic
    c.   Mydriatic agents
    d.   All of the above

57. Which route is usually used for vaccination??
    a. IV route
    b. Inhalation
    c. Oral route
    d. Intradermal

58. Which route is the slowest?
    a. Inhalation
    b. Transdermal
    c. Oral
    d. Intramuscular

59. If a patient is vomiting and cannot take a medication, or if a medication needs to be administered
    in a way that avoids the GI tract, the medication can be given:
    a. Orally
    b. Sublingually
    c. Bucally
    d. Rectally

60. Which route carries the risk of introducing pathogens into the patient's body?
    a. IV
    b. Oral
    c. Transdermal
    d. No routes are dangerous

61. It is important to do which of the following?
    a. Communicate with the patient
    b. Answer questions to the best of your ability
    c. Protect the patient's privacy

d. All of the above

62. A medication that regulates the heartbeat affects:
    a. The circulatory system
    b. The integumentary system
    c. The endocrine system
    d. The urinary tract

63. A patient is given a medication. A little while later her heart rate increases. This is a:
    a. Physiological change
    b. Psychological change
    c. Emotional change
    d. None of the above

64. A patient begins to hear things. This is a:
    a. Physiological change
    b. Psychological change
    c. Emotional change
    d. None of the above

65. Which of the following is not a word for taking medication by mouth?
    a. Oral
    b. Sublingual
    c. Parenteral
    d. Entereal

66. Which of the following should be asked for medication history?
    a. Previous medications
    b. Current medications
    c. Supplements
    d. All of the above

67. A patient tells you that he is allergic to a medication. You should ask which of the following?
    a. What kind of reaction did you have to it?
    b. What other medications are you on?
    c. What supplements are you on?
    d. Do you have a living will?

68. A patient tells you that she take supplements. You should ask:
    a. What other medications are you on?
    b. Which specific supplements do you take?
    c. Why do you take supplements?
    d. Do you have a living will?

69. Which of the following should you ask a patient for a drug history?
    a. How often do you exercise?

b. Who can I release you medical information to?

c. Are you on any vitamins?

d. How long have you had this medical complaint?

70. A patient tells you that he is on Prozac. You should ask:

    a. How often do you participate in hobbies?

    b. Do your family members react to any medications?

    c. When did you eat your last meal?

    d. What dosage of Prozac do you take?

71. A patient tells you that she is no longer on any medications due to diet and exercise. You should ask:

    a. What kind of exercise do you enjoy?

    b. Why are you visiting the hospital today?

    c. What medications have you taken in the past?

    d. What kind of vegetables do you eat?

72. You check a patient's chart and notice that he is on two medications for the same thing. This is called:

    a. Redundancy

    b. Route

    c. Right

    d. Reciprocity

73. You are supposed to give a patient a medication. You have the medication with you, but need to check the dose. Where do you find this?

    a. Patient's bracelet

    b. Chart

    c. Nurse's desk

    d. Audio files

74. You have made an error. You should:

    a. Notify your supervisor

    b. Notify the nurse/doctor

    c. Document the incident

    d. All of the above

75. Which route is the most common, safest, and economical way to administer medication?

    a. IV

    b. Oral

    c. Intramuscular

    d. Rectal

76. Medications that affect the adrenal cortex include:

    a. Hydrocortisone, and fludrocortisone.

b. Dexamethasone

c. Hydrocortisone sodium succinate

d. All of the above

77. A medication that affects breathing is said to affect:
   a. Respiratory system
   b. Nervous system
   c. Endocrine system
   d. Integumentary system

78. A medication that affects hormones and glands producing hormones is said to affect:
   a. Respiratory system
   b. Nervous system
   c. Endocrine system
   d. Integumentary system

79. A patient is on a medication to reduce stomach acid. This affects:
   a. Digestive tract
   b. Urinary tract
   c. Endocrine system
   d. Respiratory tract

80. A patient is on a medication aimed at drawing fluid away from the body tissues. This drug is a:
   a. Anticholinergic
   b. Beta blocker
   c. Amphetamine
   d. Diuretic

81. Which route can be as fast as the IV route?
   a. Inhalation
   b. Transdermal
   c. Oral
   d. Intramuscular

82. A patient tells you that he has never taken any medications other than the occasional antibiotic. You should ask:
   a. What is your complaint today?
   b. Do you exercise regularly?
   c. Do you take any vitamins or supplements?
   d. Are you sure that you are ill?

83. Where would you find the doctor's orders?
   a. The nurse's station
   b. The patient's bracelet
   c. The chart

d. Medical record's department

84. Which of the following may affect a medication taken orally?
    a. Level of stomach acid
    b. Whether or not the patient has eaten
    c. Whether or not a medication has a protective coating
    d. All of the above

85. Which of the following is essential to being a successful MT?
    a. Confidentiality
    b. Good hygiene
    c. Respect for the patient
    d. All of the above

86. You know that a certain medication has certain side effects. You should:
    a. Communicate the effects to the patient
    b. Don't say anything
    c. Give the patient a second medication to mitigate the side effects
    d. Don't give anyone that medication

87. A patient must continue a medication after she gets home. Which is the easiest way for the patient to take the medication?
    a. Intravenously
    b. Orally
    c. Subdermally
    d. Rectally

88. Which of the following is true about supplements?
    a. They do not interfere with medications
    b. They are placebos
    c. They can interact with medications
    d. They have no real effect on the human body

89. What should you do as soon as you enter a patient's room?
    a. Wash your hands
    b. Administer the medication
    c. Nothing
    d. Wait for the nurse

90. The normal range of respiration for adults is .....
    a. 5-10
    b. 12-20
    c. 25-40
    d. 30-50

91. A chemical coating that dissolves only in the upper intestine is called:
    a. Enteric coating
    b. Polycephorous coating
    c. Medical coating
    d. None of the above

92. Enteric coatings are useful for:
    a. Administering medications sublingually
    b. Protecting drugs from stomach acid
    c. Protecting drugs from teeth
    d. Administering medications intravenously

93. In order to prevent medication errors you should:
    a. Check the dosage
    b. Check the concentration
    c. Check the spelling of the medication
    d. All of the above

94. A medication technician should not:
    a. Change the dosage of a medication
    b. Administer medication orally
    c. Check the patient's chart
    d. Talk to a patient

95. A patient tells you that she is on an ophthalmic medication. This medication affects:
    a. The eyes
    b. The nose
    c. The stomach
    d. The ears

96. In order to prevent medication errors you should:
    a. Wash your hands
    b. Leave the chart alone
    c. Compare the name on the bracelet and the medication
    d. Let the patient take his own medicine

97. A patient is on a laxative. This type of medication _____
    a. Causes a patient to have frequent bowel movement.
    b. Causes constipation.
    c. Reduces pain.
    d. Causes urination.

98. You have made an error. You should:
    a. Notify your supervisor
    b. Notify the nurse/doctor
    c. Document the incident

d. All of the above

99. A medication that is administered through the spinal cord is_____
   a. IV
   b. Oral
   c. Intrathecal
   d. Rectal

100.   A medication that is absorbed through the skin is called:
   a. Oral medication
   b. Intravenous medication
   c. Topical medication
   d. Antibiotics

Section One Medication Aide Answers

1. C
2. A
3. D
4. A
5. C
6. A
7. D
8. C
9. D
10. B
11. B
12. A
13. A
14. B
15. C
16. D
17. A
18. D
19. A
20. C
21. B
22. D
23. B
24. A
25. C
26. D
27. B
28. B
29. D
30. A
31. C
32. B
33. A
34. C
35. A
36. C
37. A
38. B
39. B
40. C
41. D

42. A
43. A
44. D
45. B
46. C
47. A
48. C
49. B
50. D
51. A
52. B
53. A
54. C
55. B
56. C
57. D
58. B
59. C
60. A
61. C
62. B
63. D
64. B
65. C
66. A
67. D
68. D
69. D
70. D
71. D
72. A
73. C
74. B
75. A
76. C
77. D
78. A
79. C
80. D
81. D
82. A
83. B
84. A
85. B
86. B
87. D

88. A
89. A
90. B
91. A
92. D
93. B
94. A
95. B
96. C
97. B
98. A
99. C
100.   D

Section Two Medication Aide Answers

1. D
2. A
3. D
4. C
5. D
6. D
7. D
8. B
9. C
10. B
11. B
12. A
13. C
14. C
15. B
16. C
17. D
18. B
19. D
20. D
21. A
22. C
23. B
24. B
25. C

26. D
27. A
28. B
29. C
30. A
31. B
32. A
33. C
34. D
35. D
36. C
37. C
38. D
39. D
40. A
41. A
42. C
43. D
44. C
45. C
46. A
47. D
48. A
49. D
50. D
51. A
52. B
53. A
54. B
55. D
56. D
57. D
58. C
59. D
60. A
61. D
62. A
63. A
64. B
65. C

66. D
67. A
68. B
69. C
70. D
71. C
72. A
73. B
74. D
75. B
76. D
77. A
78. C
79. A
80. D
81. A
82. C
83. C
84. D
85. D
86. A
87. B
88. C
89. A
90. B
91. A
92. B
93. D
94. A
95. A
96. C
97. A
98. D
99. C
100.   C

OTHER TITLES FROM THE SAME AUTHOR:

1. Work At Home Jobs For Nurses & Other Healthcare Professionals

2. Nurses' Romance Series

3. CNA Exam Prep: Nurse Assistant Practice Test Questions. Vol. One and Two

4. Patient Care Technician Exam Review Questions: PCT Test Prep

5. CNA Study Guide

6. Medical Assistant Test Preparation

7. EKG Technician Study Guide

8. Phlebotomy Test Prep Vol 1, 2, & 3

9. The Home Health Aide Textbook

10. Medical Assistant Certification Study Guide Vol 1 & 2

And Many More Books

Visit www.janejohn-nwankwo.com

Search Jane John-Nwankwo on Amazon for over 50 books

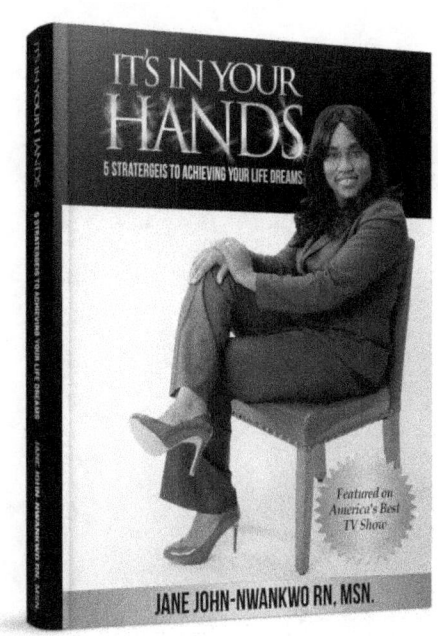

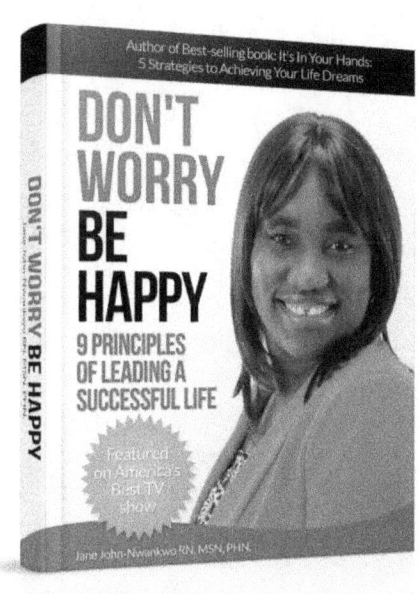

Buy on amazon.com